Buddy the Bear

"My Best Friend"

By Andrew Katz

ISBN-13: 9798867481599

From the Author

I am a totally optimistic and determined individual, but the driving forces behind me during this entire ordeal was my Wife, my Sister, my 2 Sons and Daughter in law.
I Love You & Thank You

Every story has a beginning and this is mine.

I believe that there is a time in everyone's life that you had a Teddy Bear of some shape, color or size. I know I did and I named him Joey.

Joey was "My Best Friend" that I could share stories, dreams, make wishes and also tell him my most intimate secrets because "My Best Friend" Joey would never repeat them to anyone.

Joey was part of the Italian side of our family so he had plenty of loud social skills and more importantly, he knew how to keep secrets.

Of course, high school and college came around and we couldn't have all of the conversations we once had. All and all, Joey was still "My Best Friend" and he still kept all of our secrets a secret.

I can assure you that Joey was never lonely. My Mother always introduced him to the new little family members and all of the new little kids in the neighborhood.

Joey got to play more games, meet more little friends and God only knows how many more secrets he had to keep! "My Best Friend" Joey became a "Best Friend" to many more kids.

Eventually my Mother couldn't find any more replacement parts. Joey got thinner, had one eye, one ear and a pushed in nose that interfered with his sense of smell.

Joey knew it was time to move on. My Mother made sure he moved on with dignity?

And so "my" story begins!

On the way home after surgery and an overnight stay at the hospital, my wife had to pick up a prescription from the pharmacy.

Still somewhat groggy, I impatiently waited in the car when all of a sudden, I felt the presence of something near my window. I turned, the door opened and a bear was staring me in the face. All I could say was "What the heck is that?"

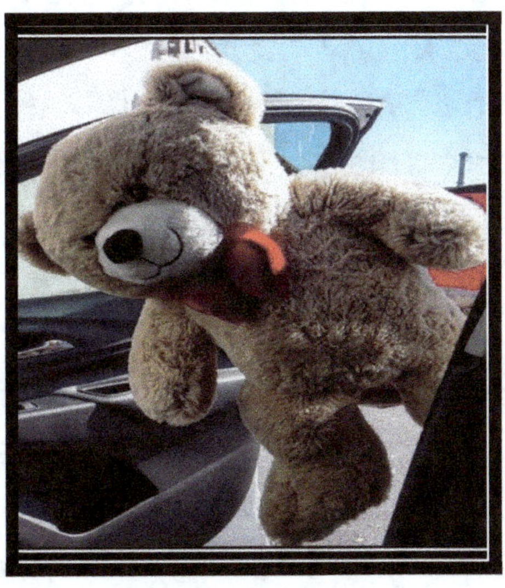

My wife said "I got you a buddy to keep you company while recuperating and going through 6 weeks of treatments." He called to me when I was walking down the aisle to the pharmacy and he smiled at me when I passed him on the way back to the checkout!"

After putting the bear on my lap and getting in the car she said, "What was I to do? He was telling me to take him home and besides, now you have a buddy to watch over you at night!"

And now you know how and why he was named Buddy the Bear and he was going to be "My Best Friend". "And just think about this for a moment. I am only 75 years old?????"

Well, Buddy had no idea what he was in for in his new home. He was going to learn a lot about life, how it works and why it works. He will also learn respect, manners, how to be self-sufficient and that's only on his first day! (*only kidding*)

Needless to say, we haven't had anyone under the age of 40 in our home for quite some time, let alone a bear that is intended to be "My Best Friend".

The first order of business coming up was a Birthday Party for my wife and you will never guess who showed up first and was dressed for the occasion? He just couldn't help himself.

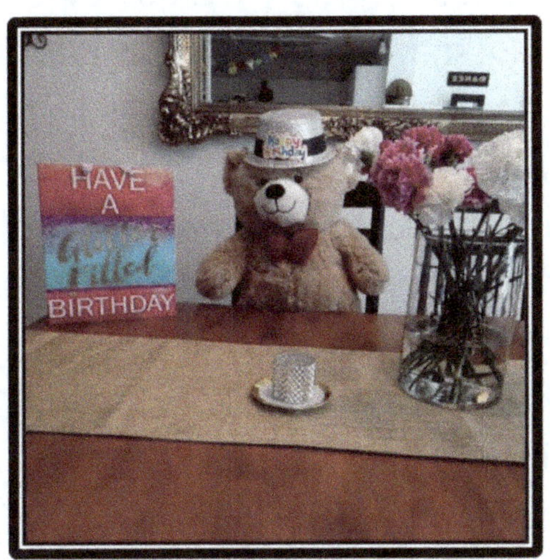

The party was a reminder that recoup from surgery was completed now and in 2 weeks I would have to start the weekly regiment of 6 weeks straight of treatment.

The days between the party and my treatments starting on Wednesday gave

Buddy and me time to talk about life. We always waited until bedtime when the house was totally quiet.

Buddy didn't know how to talk yet but he was a great listener and I could tell him all of the things that were on my mind. I even told him about Joey and I think the smile on his face got bigger.

I also knew that Buddy wouldn't tell anyone about our conversations because he was "My Best Friend". In fact, I think he enjoyed it because it was probably better than one of my bedtime stories.

I told him about all of the things I wanted him to learn and I was going to teach him just like I did Joey.

I think I saw him shake his head in approval. In fact, I believed he already knew a lot. He was just going to have to think it through and make a decision about what he wanted.

After all, do bears adjust to our domesticated lifestyle or do they need to be in the wild?

Well, tomorrow is another day and "My Best Friend" had a lot of thinking to do.

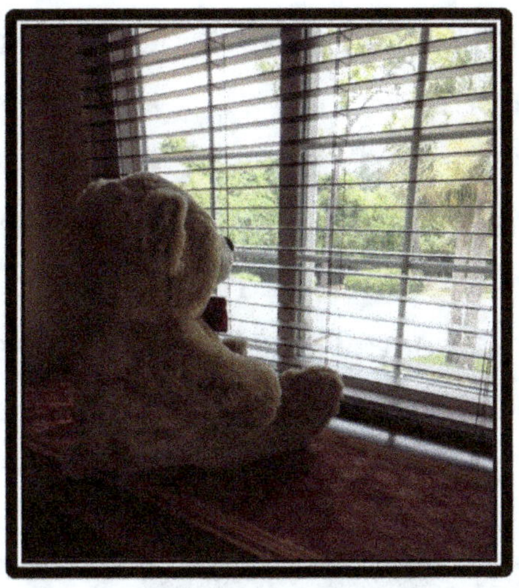

That night when it was all quiet again, we talked and I let him know my treatments started tomorrow. I also told him that the couple of days after would not be easy.

I didn't mention anything about our conversation the night before, but I let him know I couldn't talk very long because tomorrow would be here before you know it. I rolled over and all of sudden I heard this little gruff voice. "Good Night Dad." (??)

The next morning, I told my wife what happened and she just smiled. We had our coffee and got ourselves ready to go because I couldn't be late for my appointment.

We locked up, went to the garage, got in the car and I couldn't believe my eyes. In the back seat with that smug look on his face was "My Best Friend" and I knew at that moment he had decided to stay.

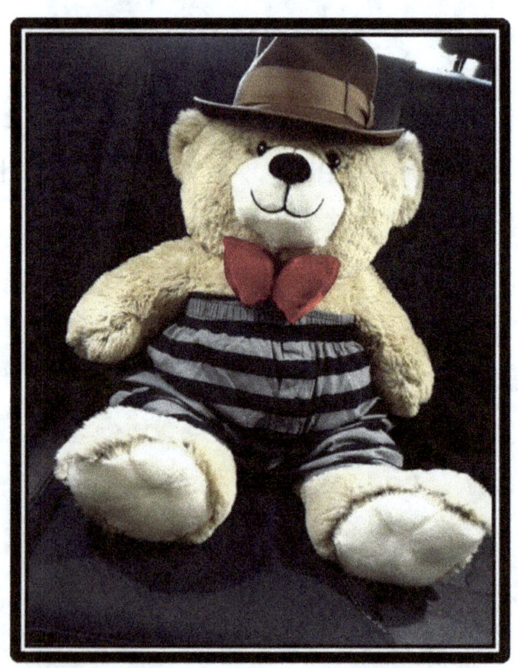

My wife just smiled letting me
know she got him dressed and in
the car because she already knew that
he wanted to go. Leave it to a woman's
intuition!

It was the first trip for treatment
and only 5 more to go. Can't
wait? The day of and the day after are
quite difficult but after that, Buddy and
I can hang out together for 5 days until
the next treatment.

I promised him I would teach him
like I did Joey and I still believed Buddy
already knew quite a bit and a lot more
than he was letting on.

Besides that, I know he can talk
and it makes me wonder if anyone else
can hear him when he does. I would have
to guess it would be my wife!

When I get home from treatment,
I have a rotation cycle on all four sides
of my body for 2 hours and flat on my
stomach is the most uncomfortable.

My wife came in the bedroom with
Buddy and said he wanted to keep me

company. And what a surprise it was when she put him on the floor in front of me and he started reading out loud in his little gruff voice. "How did she know? I wonder"!

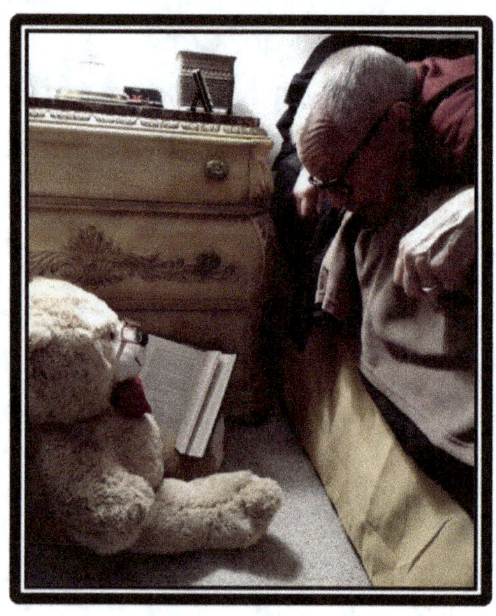

At this rate we should be able to read the Sunday newspaper together while we have a cup of coffee. I think Buddy will drink coffee? After all, he is always surprising me with things I didn't know he could do, would do or even say?

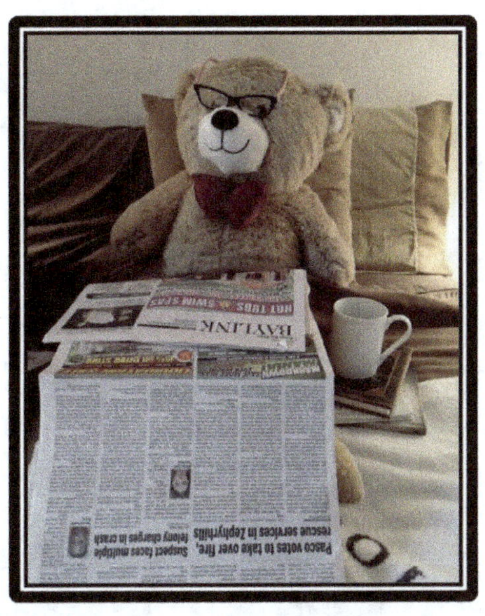

He was growing up pretty quick and the five more weeks of treatments would give us time to learn more about each other. Buddy has become part of our family and he definitely is "My Best Friend".

By treatment no.2 my wife moved her sleeping quarters to the guest bedroom because I get up and down all night long and there wasn't any reason for her to be awake all night. After all, she had to take on all of the household responsibilities that we shared before this started.

That left Buddy to keep watch over me. He went everywhere that we had to go and he even started wearing a mask to protect me from any COVID virus exposure that was currently happening in the world.

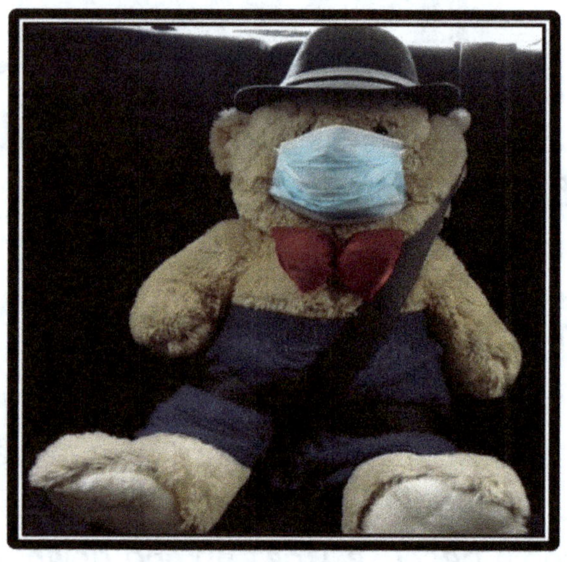

At night I talked to him about everything that was going on in our lives. He knew I was concerned about what would happen if things worked out in our

favor and also what would happen if they
didn't. He is such a good listener.

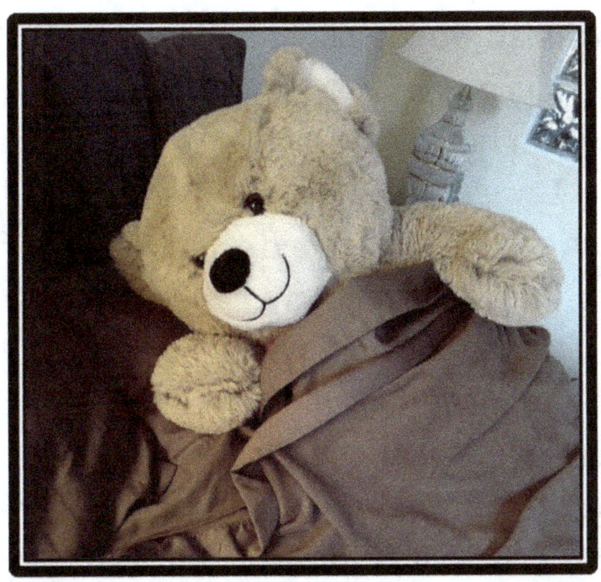

He would just lay there and look at
me with that smile on his face and I
swear I could hear him say in his little
gruff voice, "Don't worry Dad, everything
will be okay, I promise."
The next day my wife had some
errands to run plus the grocery shopping.
She mentioned it would be a while, but
Buddy would be here to watch out for me

and I should keep an eye on him since he has started to crawl.

On her way out the door she mentioned Buddy again because he had also figured out how to get down the stairs on his butt.

I was having a really bad day and I dozed off until I heard this little gruff voice in the back of my head saying "Dad, are you okay? Dad, are you okay?" It startled me out of a deep sleep. I looked around the room and Buddy was nowhere in sight. I got up and checked the other rooms and still no Buddy. "Maybe I was just dreaming".

I decided to check downstairs. I got down the first 2 flights, turned the corner and who do you think I saw? Buddy "trying" to get up the steps to see if I was okay?

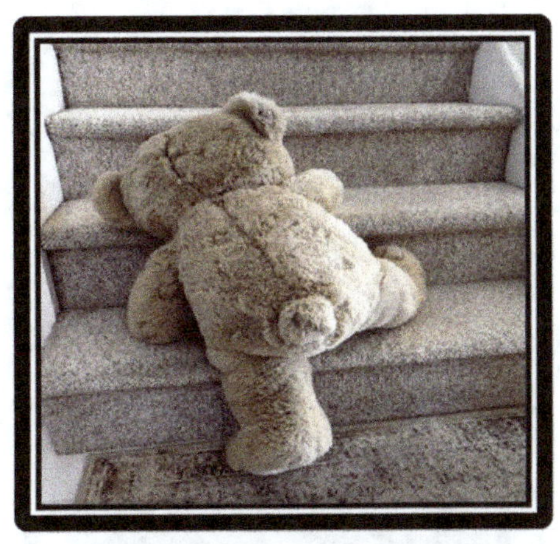

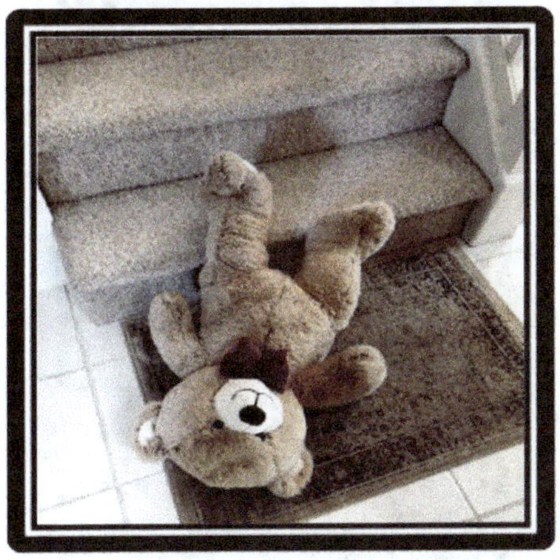

Think that's' a bad day? At that moment, my wife walked in the door and you would never guess who was in trouble? Starts with an **M** and ends with an **E**!!!

By the time the 4th treatment was approaching Buddy was learning to walk and not the easy way.

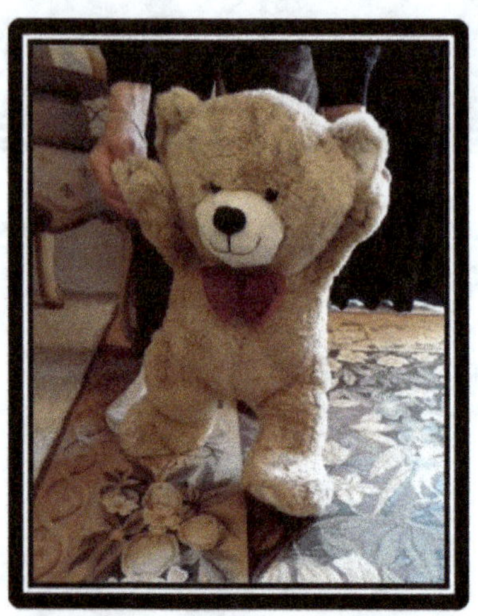

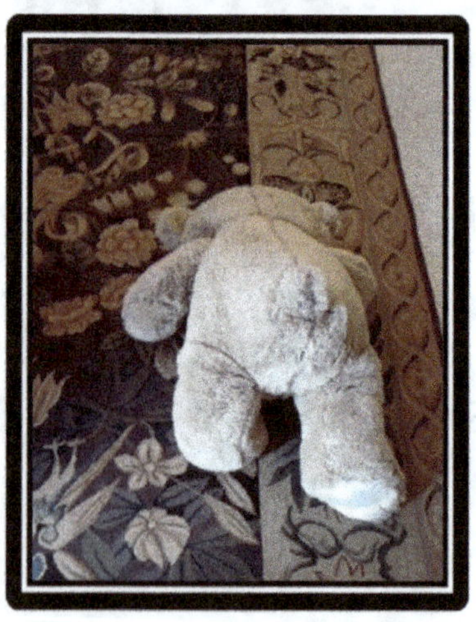

One night after the lights were out, Buddy asked me if he was doing a good job watching out for me and was he still "My Best Friend"?

I told him that he was the most awesome best friend a person could have and I'm so glad Mom picked him out to come home with us. "In fact Buddy, we are both happy that you are in our family."

Buddy said in his little gruff voice? "Thanks Dad, that makes me feel really good. Good night and I want to learn how to drive so I can take you for treatments?" I rolled my eyes, turned over and shook my head "Yessiree", no hands and no legs to speak of and he wanted to drive?"

The next morning was trash day so I went out to the garage to take the containers to the curb and what do you think I saw? The garage door was open, the car was gone and who was in the driveway???

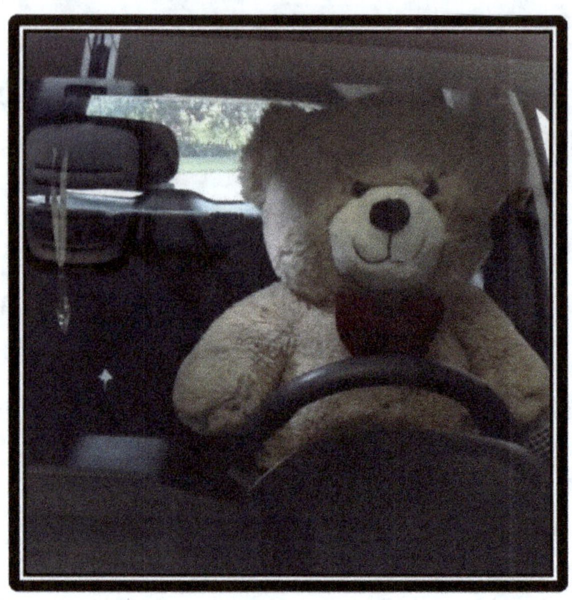

I certainly hope that my wife was involved in this, but I am almost afraid to ask?

Finally, the 6th and last treatment came and of course Buddy didn't drive and all of us can thank our "lucky stars" for that.

Everyone was ready for this to be over and personally I was way over ready. Now we can hopefully have some sort of normalcy back in our lives for at least 6 weeks while everything heals inside. Then it will be back for a checkup

and we are hopeful that everything will
be fine.

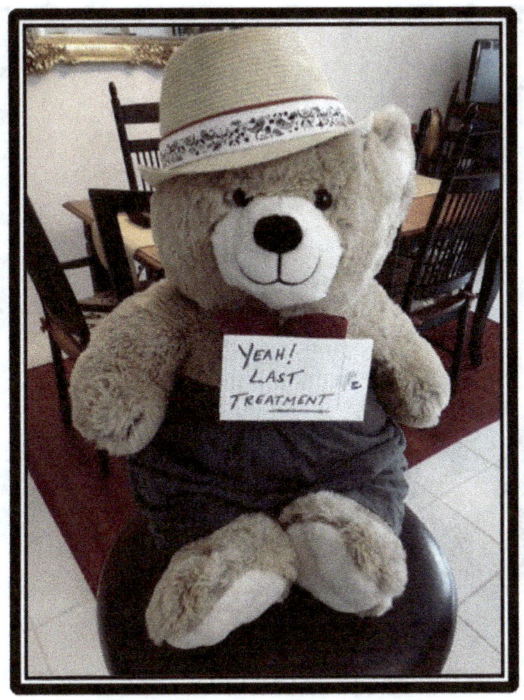

With 6 weeks of freedom, we
wanted to have some fun and enjoy the
time until then.

Buddy was more than ready and the
first thing he wanted to do was dress
like everyone else, so off to the mall we
went. It's not easy finding clothes that

will fit a bear, but we did the best we could.

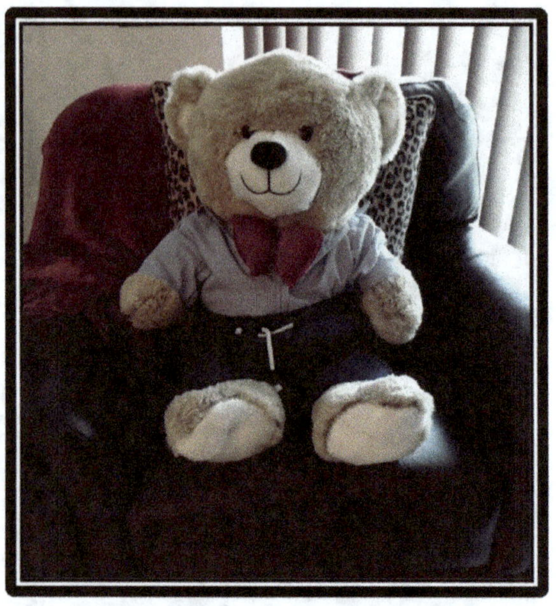

That nasty Covid Virus was still in the U.S. and everyone had to wear a mask in public.

When the restrictions were lifted a little, we traveled 200 miles so Buddy could meet his only Aunt.

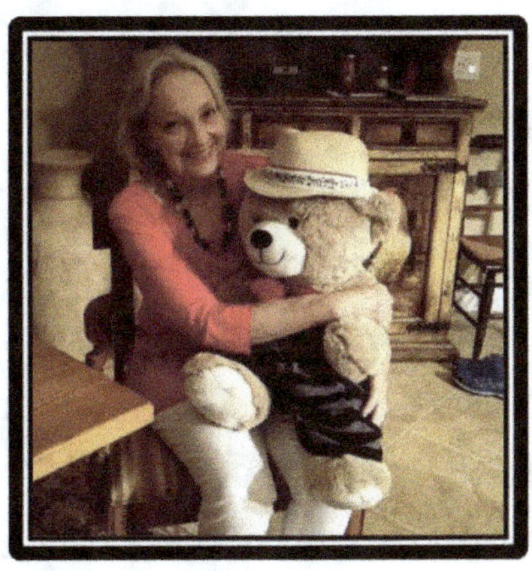

We returned home a few days before my scheduled checkup. It gave Buddy and me some time to talk when the lights were out and the house was quiet.

The night before the checkup he did have a question? He wanted to know what would happen to him if something happened to me. So, I told him he would have to put up with Mom. ("Oops, did I just say that?") haha

I told him he would be lucky to have Mom because she is a lot more compassionate than I am. He just shook his head up and down and I swear he rolled his eyes with a smart aleck expression that said ("Yes, I certainly know that!")

It was also the moment and the look on his face that I think he would have had tears in his eyes if he was able? And then I said, "Don't worry Buddy, because regardless of what happens, you will always be "My Best Friend" and he smiled.

Well, the checkup didn't go as well as we thought it would. Surgery was scheduled for the following week with an overnight stay and Buddy was not very happy.

Even worse, the morning when we had to leave he was waiting at the front door and I had to tell him that bears were not allowed in the Hospital.

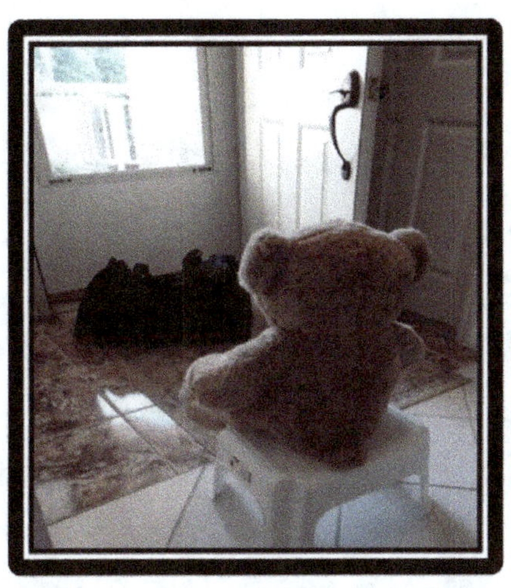

A few days later we received the news. The results from the biopsy were not good and there were decisions that had to be made? There was a lot that my wife and I would have to think about and talk about after we wrap our heads around the issues.

We have always talked everything through, but this issue has a lot more negatives to overcome.

And of course, after my wife and I have reached our decisions, I will wait until the lights are out and everything is quiet to have a discussion with Buddy. After all, he is "My Best Friend".

Just so you know,

This story is about Cancer returning after 10 years and returning aggressively. Mine is in the bladder.

There are many emotions involved in wrapping our heads around it all. Thank goodness for a great and strong husband and wife relationship with a lot of love. Our family is quite small but gigantic in love and support.

My wife and I have always worked together as a team. It takes many conversations, multiple decisions and planning ahead. This time will be more crucial than ever. In fact, we always plan for the worst and we will always hope for the best!

This brings me to the point and my reason for telling you about Buddy the Bear, "My Best Friend".

The day my wife found Buddy while going to the pharmacy after my first surgery, little did we know, he would turn out to be the best medicine we could have purchased that day!

As you have probably realized, we both have mastered his little gruff voice and he has mastered getting the two of us through this process. Buddy picks me up when I am down and Buddy picks my wife up when she is down.

I cannot tell you the laughs that we have had with Buddy and I hope that reading this will make you laugh too. It is amazing what a Bear did for me as a child and what it can do for adults going through the process of life.

"Thanks Mom, for my bear Joey when I was a little boy" and at 75 years old "Thanks to my wife for Buddy "My Best Friend". It's was all in the timing?

And now for the rest of the story.

The Urologist recommended a treatment that I could qualify for and it is quite intense but it had a success rate of 60%? If I made the 60%, I could get another 2 to 5 years. Maybe? The only other alternative was to remove the prostate and bladder, go through Chemotherapy and Radiation and you know what happens sooner than later.

We would have to see an Oncologist and a Radiologist. Perfect, just what we wanted to hear?

Just so you know my wife and I are aware that regardless of what we try it will never cure my Cancer. It will only give us more time. We both know and realize what the inevitable is.

We may not like it, but everyone has to face and accept things that they may not like. With that being said, we decided to give this treatment a shot and if it doesn't work, then so be it.

My body will have to endure 6 weeks of Chemo and Radiation simultaneously. Chemotherapy is 1 week, 5 days in a row with 4 weeks off and another week 5 days in a row again and Chemo will be completed. Radiation is 5 days a week for the entire 6 weeks even during Chemo.

Before we start, I will also have to have a Port installed for the Chemo so back to you know where? Yep, the Hospital! I am now considered a regular where everybody knows my name.

With the decision made, we have the weekend to prepare and celebrate another family Birthday.

That night when the lights were out and the house was quiet, I let Buddy know that I would have to go to the hospital again, but just for a Day Surgery. It was only a procedure to have a Port put in for the Chemo portion of the treatments.

With the Port I can spend 5 hours the 1st day of Chemo at the clinic and the remaining 4 days I would have a battery pack loaded with Chemo and timer, about 4 to 5 ft. of tubing and a fanny pack to have the Chemo administered throughout the day. That includes while I am having Radiation.

I let Buddy know I would be home every day so he could watch out for me. That was the good news. The bad news, I also had to let him know that with the Covid virus still running rampant he couldn't go with us tomorrow.

He also couldn't go to the Doctors or to the Hospital or the Clinic for Chemo or for my daily Radiation treatments which will begin 2 days after my Port is installed. You can only imagine how that conversation went.

He was sad and I think his eyes began to water, but he didn't say a word. I knew he was disappointed. After all, he was "My Best Friend", I was his Best Friend and I knew what he was thinking? My wife put him in charge of watching out for me, but how can he do that when he isn't allowed to go anywhere that I have to go?

Monday morning we had the final meeting with the Oncologist to discuss the details on the type of Chemotherapy that they would use and what to expect.

Following that meeting we had to meet with the Radiologist for a CT scan and some kind of fitting so they could target the tumor areas and decide how they would approach them.

They were also going to discuss the diet I would have to start immediately and that would mean no gassy foods including peanut butter, no foods containing fiber including Metamucil, no drinks that are carbonated and nothing with whole grain.

Oh No!!! No more Cheerios for breakfast???

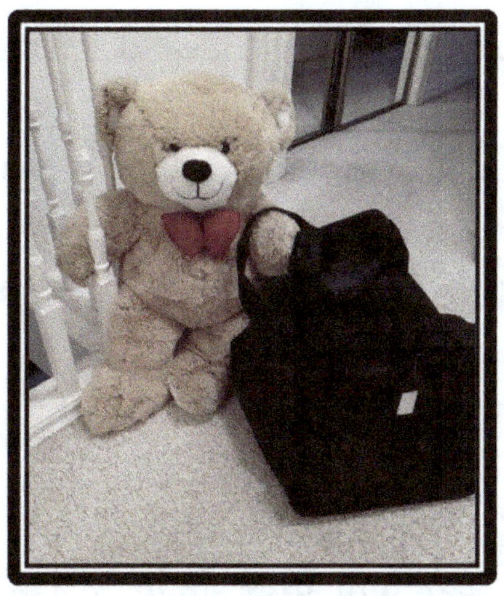

Well, guess who was in the hallway as we were heading down the stairs to get to my appointments? With his little gruff voice he said, "If I can't be your "Best Friend" and watch out for you like Mom wanted me to, then there isn't any reason for me to be here. There are plenty of people that could use a Best Friend. I love you I will miss you and Bye."

By the way, "Could you give me a ride and drop me off anywhere so I can find a new home and a "new" Best Friend!"

"I swear I could see a tear as he spoke"?

My wife replied, "I will take you anywhere that you want to go with one condition. You will have to wait until we get back from our scheduled appointments. We can't miss any of them."

"We love you too Buddy and we will miss you. We will just have to find another bear to watch over Dad!" Buddy just stood there in amazement?

We weren't concerned. Have you ever seen a bear 26 inches tall with only 8 inch long arms try to reach a doorknob?

He is stubborn and he will try and I think he gets that from my wife????

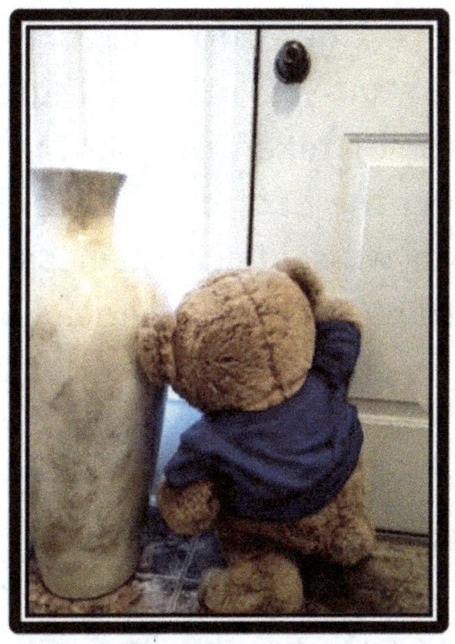

By the time we got home all was well with Buddy. He had several hours to think about it and it was safe to assume he reconsidered. "I think the doorknob reach discouraged him!"

The next couple of days went by rather quickly and I was on my way to have the Port put in so I could start my Chemo Monday morning and start Radiation on Tuesday morning.

Before I get into this part of our journey, I want you to know that my wife and I have not taken this lightly, we are just making the best of it.

After we sold our business, my wife supervised a Cardiology medical office for 9 years and I volunteered in a Hospital Emergency Room. It was an invaluable education in life and death for the both of us, especially now.

My wife actually had her first experience with death when she lost her Mother to Breast and Bone Cancer at a very young age. It was all of these things, combined with our understanding of the human life cycle that made "some" of this a little easier to handle mentally.

We also realize that a lot of things are not our choice? I always said "it was the "luck of the draw" or better said; "it is in the cards we were dealt when we entered at birth". We just don't get to see them until they are dealt to us one at a time." This card was like "WOW" what has just happened and why now?

Even worse, all of a sudden we became one of the couples we had met and observed as they went through the process. Now we were on their side of the window and I had the life threatening disease that was going to change our lives and all of the plans we had made together.

At that moment, all of the things we had worked towards were flushed, right down the toilet.

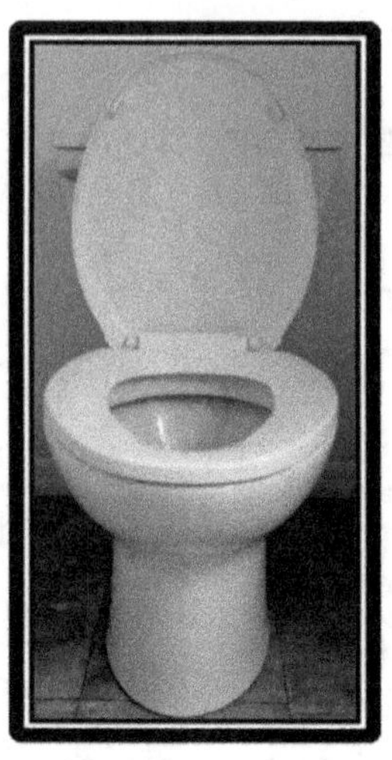

Now let's talk about the Port and the fun that we had? Friday, we arrived on time and again it was at the Hospital I volunteer at, so of course everybody knows my name and even better, I know theirs. It made for a much more comfortable visit for me mentally, if there is such a thing as comfortable when experiencing an unknown.

In case you were thinking it, I wasn't getting preferential treatment. I was getting the same treatment that any other patient would. It's one of the reasons that I feel proud to be a part of the team on the days I volunteer. It makes me feel good.

Anyway, I had to undress, give blood and speak with the Doctor explaining the process, (Yada Yada & Yada).

Just think, I only had to be there 2 hours ahead of time for a procedure that was going to take 30 minutes. That 30 minutes included the prep, hook ups with oxygen and the 10 minutes to cut, insert a Port with a tube going to a vein in my neck, a few stitches, instructions and out to recovery.

I also think there was a timing contest going on for that particular procedure that I wasn't aware of and I believe our team won. I could swear I heard one of the nurses click the timer on and off? (haha)

On the way home we wondered if Buddy may have had a change of heart, or was he packed and ready to leave home again? Well, we had our answer when we walked in the door.

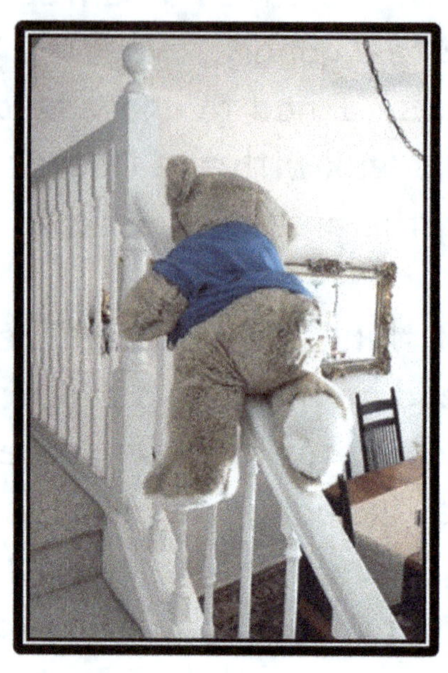

Now the excitement?

I do have to tell you that the list of do's and don'ts with the Port over the next 5 days left me speechless. It would have been a heck of a lot easier to take tap dance lessons instead!

I start Chemo Monday and Radiation on Tuesday. My first don't (and I am right-handed), I can't raise my right arm to do anything for 5 days and the second don't, I can't get the top clear bandage wet when I shower, so guess how many people it takes for one man to shower?

I know the answer. Only TWO!

My poor wife!!! "I hope she doesn't start packing her suitcases anytime soon." If she does, I will need to find the proverbial creek and look for a paddle?

Tomorrow morning, we will learn the Port dance needed to shower, wash hair and dry off. Almost forgot, I will also have to get dressed and undressed.

Sounds like my pre-Kindergarten years when someone had to help me do all of that, "Thanks again Mom".

And just think, we haven't even added the fanny pack with 4 to 5 ft of plastic tubing that will be pumping Chemo 24 hours a day. At least we will have 2 days of practice before we add the fanny pack. Talk about dancing?

It should be fairly easy. My wife just has to wash my left arm, my hair, my back and my right ear. Rinse and do not get the bandage over the Port wet???

2 days later with fanny pack attached the dance got better because she also had to hold the pack outside of the shower to prevent the tubing from pulling out of the Port and getting tangled. I would not be able to turn around. Great!!!

All I can say about sleeping with that and going to Radiation along with everyday functions is, "You've got to Be Kidding Me!" Did I mention getting dressed and undressed?

At this point, I think everyone understands the processes of Chemo and Radiation and it's fair to say it isn't much fun so we won't discuss it any longer.

There is only one thing that comes to mind at this point. "I think I really need to hide my wife's suitcases."

To make all of this even more interesting, with only two weeks left to go and after my Friday Radiation treatment we were at home eating lunch at the kitchen bar.

I had no memory of it, but I started babbling incoherently while chasing a slice of canned peach around the plate. All I wanted to do was cut it with my fork so I could eat it?

Well, I guess I didn't do a very good job of it because I passed out and my head went into the plate head first.

My wife jumped into action calling 911 while reaching in my mouth for any food that may have been stuck in my throat and proceeding to the Heimlich maneuver. She even kept me from falling on to the tile floor and cracking my head open.

When I finally opened my eyes, the first thing I saw was a Paramedic. "Surprise"!

Long story short, I had my first ambulance ride and Emergency Room visit as a patient. Now that's an exciting adventure. I couldn't have made it another day in this lifetime without the experience???

*"(I would like to mention a special thank you with a lot of love to my "Kindred Spirit" that by **"coincidence?"** happened to be working in the ER that day and I feel she was there for me and she was comforting for my wife. She made all of our scary moments disappear.)*

I was admitted into the hospital that evening and my wife had to go back home because the Covid virus was still running rampant. We talked on the phone through the night every time a test was done and when I received the results.

The next day she would be able to come in during visiting hours and hopefully this would all be behind us soon.

At home Buddy was not handling this very well.

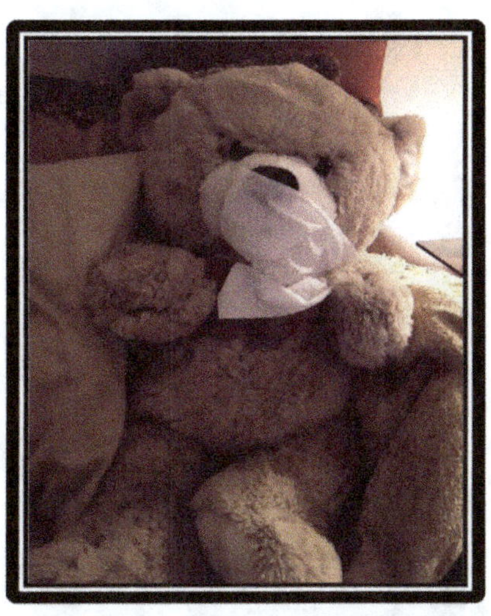

Many tests later the diagnosis in English was dehydration, diarrhea and my brain had short circuited from all that was going on in my body. It had to find center again. The "Good News", my brain didn't have to be removed?????

I was discharged that evening and we headed home. Buddy was happy about that because next weekend was Halloween and he was ready.

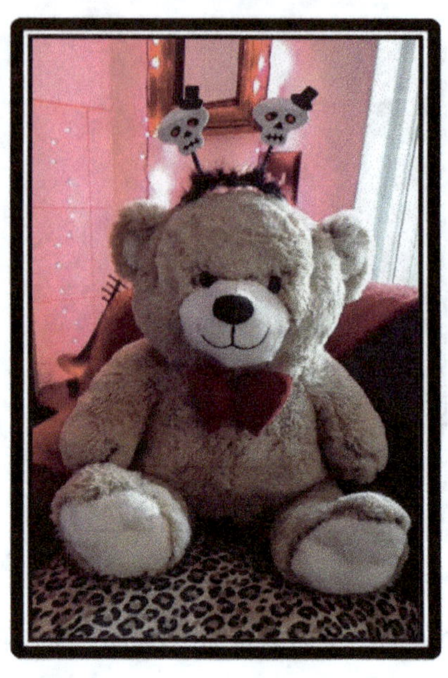

Nov 6th my treatments will be completed and I could start recouping without interruption and it wouldn't be long Santa would be loading up his sleigh, the Ball would be dropping in Times Square and this God awful year would be over.

We will have a couple follow up appointments and the week before Christmas I will have my Cystoscopy to take a look inside and find out if the treatment worked and what comes next.

That would give us plenty of time to decorate, put up the tree, plan Christmas Eve dinner and do a little shopping etc. Everything is different with this awful Covid Virus wreaking havoc in the Country, but we still love the Holidays. As a matter of fact, we are going to enjoy it and get in the Holiday spirit early.

We will even have time to play more cards and do puzzles in the evenings. We discovered through all of this that puzzles and cards are quite soothing for us and it takes our mind off of all that is happening.

Everyone finds different distractions and those just happened to work for us. Our best "Distraction" has been Buddy the Bear, "My Best Friend".

We also learned that Buddy loves Earth Wind and Fire's music. One of his favorites is Boogie Wonderland and up on the bar he went.

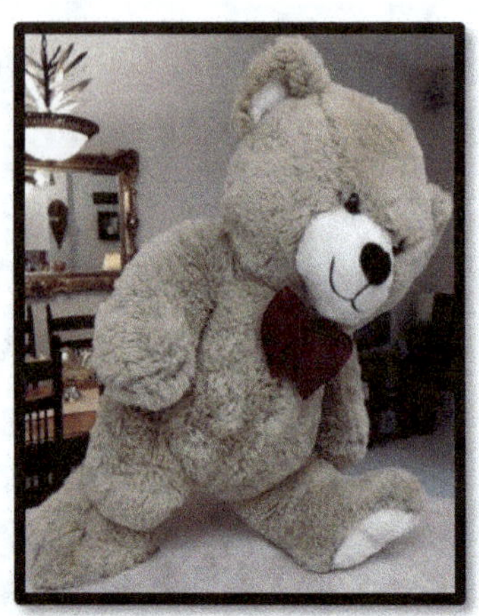

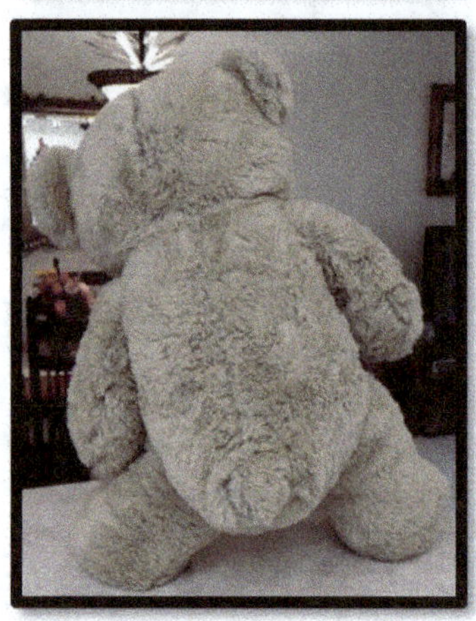

And "Boogie" he did

The week before Thanksgiving all of the decorating was done and Turkey Day arrived. Thanksgiving Day is "Pajama Day" all day for us, along with The Macy's Parade, Cinnamon Buns and a Wine toast at noon when Santa arrives.

It was a virtual parade this year without a million people lining the streets. The Covid virus has changed everything for everyone this year Worldwide, but life goes on and you make the best of it. Buddy joined us this year.

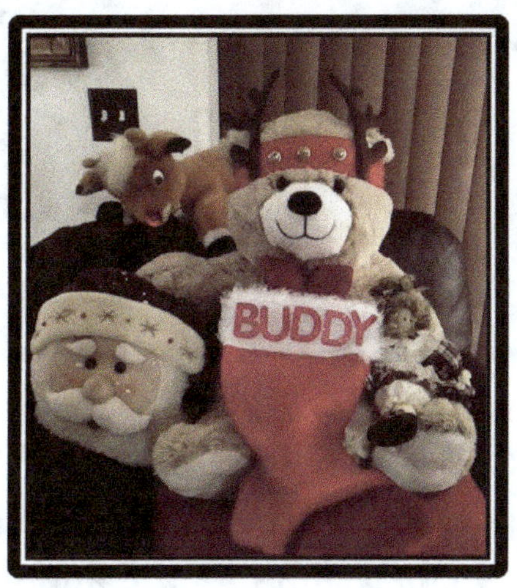

Later that day there was a knock at the door and what a surprise? Buddy had a cousin that was trying to find him and she did. She had nowhere to go and nowhere to stay. Of course, Buddy invited her in and they sat in front of the fireplace so she could warm up. "Yes, it gets cold in Florida"

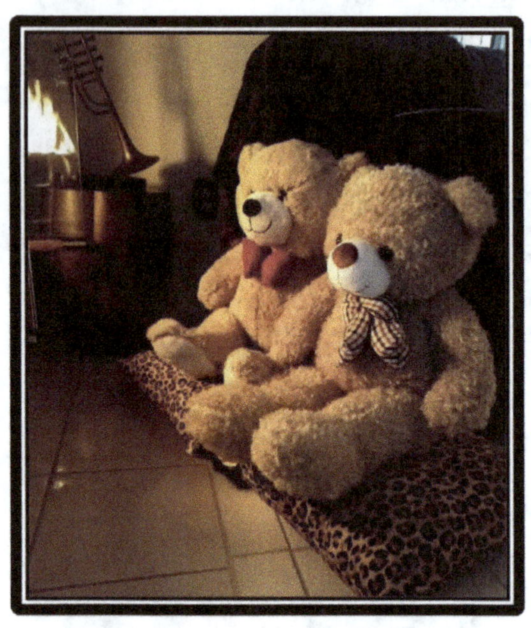

That night when the lights were out and the house was quiet, I knew Buddy had something on his mind and wanted to talk.

With his little gruff voice he said "My cousin doesn't have anywhere to go and I'm not being mean, but I don't want another bear in MY space, cousin or no cousin. And besides that, she's a girl?"

"Do you think that Aunt Gloria would like to have her as "Her Best

Friend" and she could live in her house since she lost her husband to Alzheimer's disease 4 years ago?"

"I can even train her to be a "Best Friend" before we go visit Aunt Gloria in a few weeks for her Birthday and Christmas."

"That would really surprise Aunt Gloria. Please, please Dad, can we do it?"

Go figure, Buddy thought of a way to dump his cousin and she had only been in our home a total of 8 hours!!!!

Time was clicking by and the day before my Cystoscopy appointment a package arrived from my Sister and guess what was in it? "Lucky Socks"?

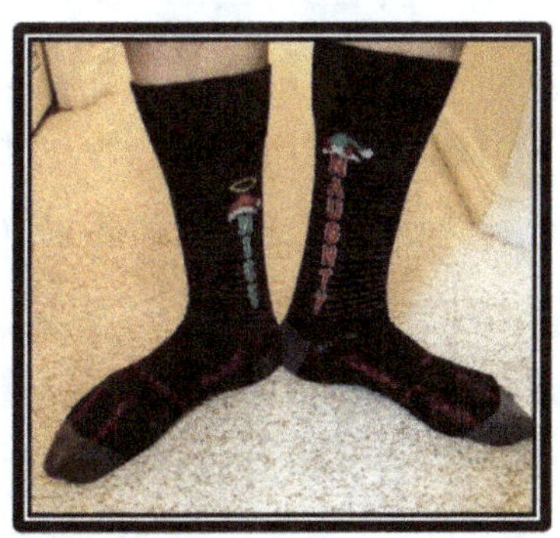

It wasn't a good night's sleep for us that night. We were too busy talking to the "Big Guy", Moms & Dads and anyone else that might have some pull.

We arrived at the Urologist's office 20 minutes early as we always do in hopes of getting in sooner. I suppose we are slow learners because it has never ever worked and it wasn't going to work on this very important nerve-racking day.

As I paced, there was one thought that went over and over in my mind since last night and I'm sure it was on my wife's mind as well since we think alike.

A 35 minute procedure which included the prep time, the Doctor's time and a scope used for this purpose that was going to determine my fate.

Was the Chemo and Radiation effective or did I go through this and put my wife and family through this for almost a whole year of Hell for nothing? Will I receive a death sentence or will I get more time?

At that very moment the Nurse called my name to come back. I hugged and kissed my wife and told her I loved her. The 25 steps or so to the door leading to the back felt more like 100 yards. I turned, looked at my wife, we waved and I went inside.

Almost like clockwork I was back in the lobby standing in front of her and I said "I don't have to come back for 3 months." We were out of there in a flash.

In the car we had our happy tears and headed home to get ready for Christmas. "I think it was the Lucky Socks?"

We don't know if it will get us 3 more months next time or if it will be one month, but we do know that we will take the time we get.

When we arrived home and told Buddy the good news he was so happy that he jumped up so high my wife had to catch him on his way back to Earth.

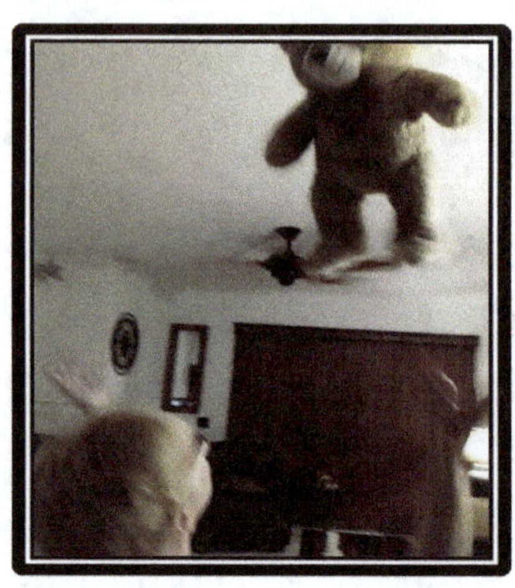

Christmas Eve was upon us and the "kids" that are in their 40's? look forward to it every year. The theme and the 4 or 5 courses of food plus a few appetizers and dessert are different every year. We eat, drink, tell stories, open gifts and just share the evening. They only stay for 6 or 7 hours?

The best part this year? "I am here to enjoy it!!!

Buddy even got a "stocking" from Santa because Santa knew that Buddy the Bear was "My Best Friend" and Buddy couldn't wait to see what was in it. In fact, we couldn't wait either.

Excited, he reached in that stocking as fast as his little arms could go to find his gift. "Teddy Grahams fit for a King"

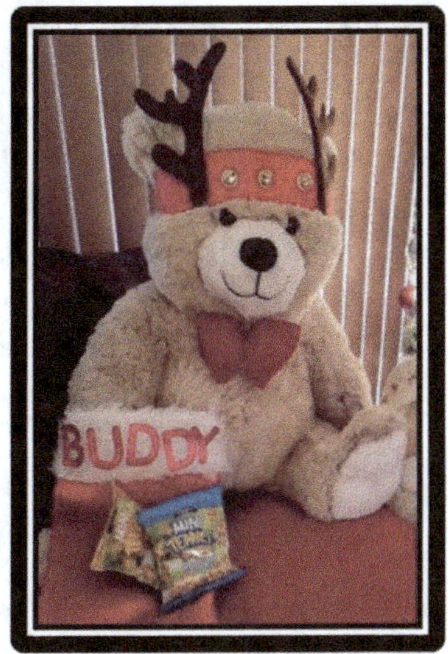

Christmas Eve rolled right into New Years Eve and before you knew it, the four of us were on our way to Aunt Gloria's house to celebrate Christmas and Birthday.

Now, in case you are wondering where his cousin is, she is in the very large red and blue bag on the floor in front of Buddy. Why??? Buddy didn't

want to share "his" back seat so he
concocted a plan?

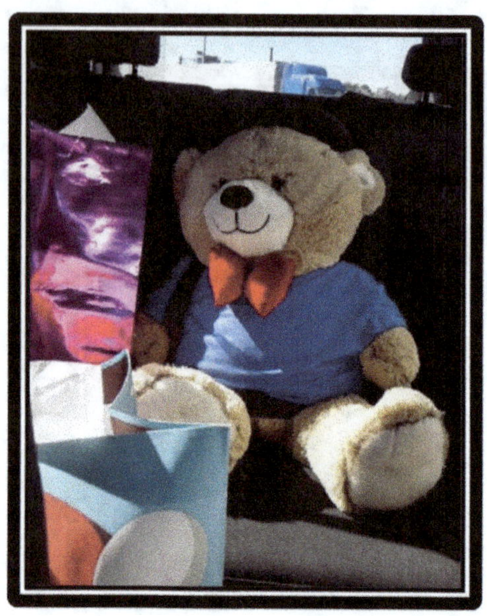

    Instead of the proverbial "Jack in
a Box" he wanted to surprise Aunt Gloria
with a "Bear in a Bag"?????
    I do have to say that Aunt Gloria
was really surprised and I also have to
say it was an emotional surprise filled
with laughter that brings tears, joy and
memories. **"Happy Birthday and Merry
Christmas Aunt Gloria"**

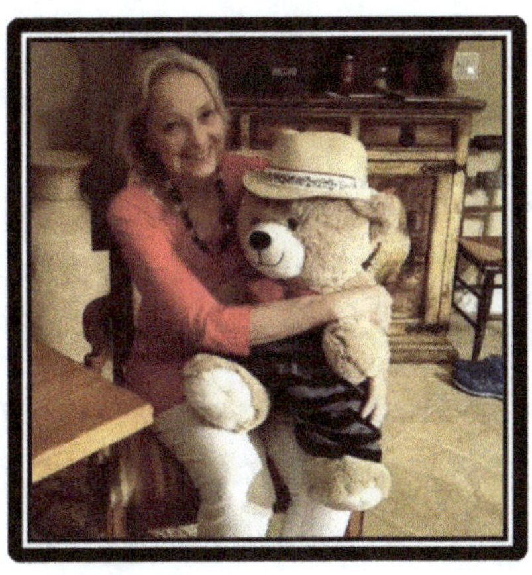

She named Buddy's cousin "Minnie"
after our Italian Grandmother. Now
Aunt Gloria had Minnie the Bear to be
her "Best Friend" and had someone to
tell all of her secrets to. Minnie will
always be there to watch out for her.

In fact, when Buddy talks to Aunt
Gloria on the phone he will able to talk to
Minnie too.

Not being able to sleep much that
night I sat in the chair next to the bed
and my thoughts turned to my sister and
brother in- law.

It was the conversations my wife
and I used to have when my sister's
husband began showing the early signs of

Dementia that progressed to Alzheimer's disease.

She had to come to the realization that the super intelligent business man she married and the beautiful life the two of them had built together would never be the same again. Her husband's brain was going to be totally destroyed. One day at a time!

She never missed a day visiting him in the ALF. Her one comforting thought through it all and to this day was their bond and their love. It was so strong, that he never forgot who she was.

Just so you know, regardless of the kind of life changing disease that is eventually going to kill the person you love, it is also going to kill a little part of you as well.

We couldn't fathom what it felt like coming home at the end of the day, every day, until this year.

My wife had to go home alone to an empty house when I had to stay in the hospital. She would share her frustration with Buddy and he would just look up and give her that reassuring smile.

I wiped the tears from my eyes, crawled back in bed and drifted off to sleep. Tomorrow, we have more celebrating to do and we all know how to do that.

We ate at restaurants and we ate at home. We enjoyed Christmas and Birthday to the max. There were times we laughed so hard we cried. We toasted everyone including those that were no longer in our lives. "They weren't in our lives, but they are always in our hearts".

While we were having our celebrations, Buddy was giving Minnie the final grand tour of the house and finishing up her training so she could be the "Best Friend" Aunt Gloria ever had. Now there will always be a smiling face for Aunt Gloria when she walks in the door.

There never seems to be enough time and we are always happy to see each other. It's also very emotional to leave, but it was time to head back home. Unfortunately, reality does exist and we all have things to do.

Between Birthday and Christmas and the time the 5 of us spent together I think that Buddy gained a totally different prospective and respect for "girls", especially his cousin Minnie.

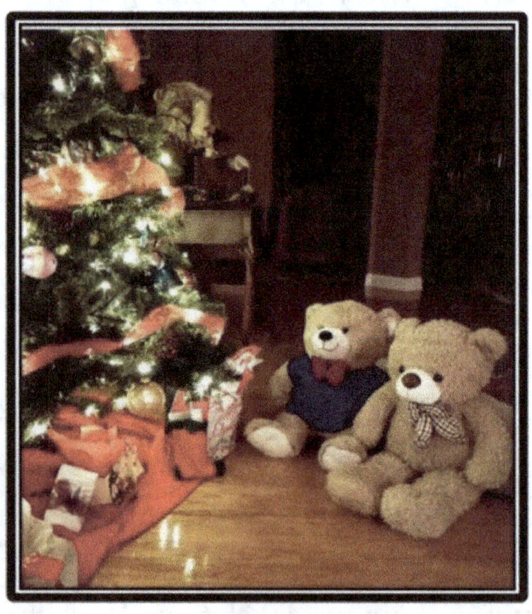

A couple of nights later when the lights were out and the house was quiet, Buddy turned and with his little gruff voice he said, "Dad, can we go up to the park tomorrow? It's only 2 blocks from here and I have some stuff I need to ask you.

I told him that if he wanted to talk now we could and he said "No, not now. It can wait until tomorrow."????

The next morning we headed up to the park and walked around the trails listening to the birds and watching the squirrels chase each other around the trees. There wasn't a cloud in the sky.

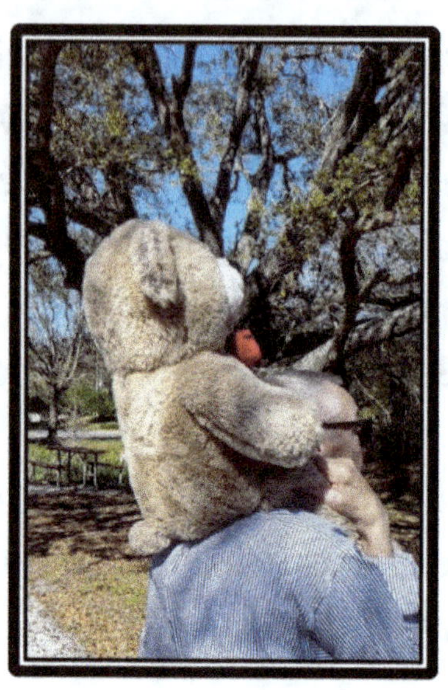

We sat down on one of the benches and Buddy looked at me and with his little gruff voice he said, "Dad, what's going to happen to me and Mom when you die? I'm your "Best Friend" and Mom said I'm supposed to watch out for you, but what will really happen to me?"

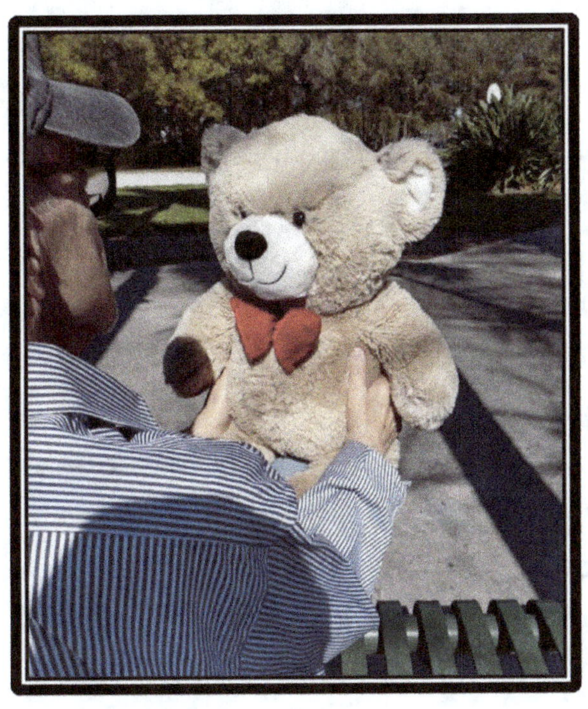

I looked at him in surprise and told him that the next person in command would have to decide that and we know who she is.

His eyes got as big as moon pies as he blurted out **"MOM?????"** Well, at least I won't have to leave home. **Will I?"**

I told him "No, you won't have to leave home Buddy. Mom will need a "Best Friend" and who better than you. I will always be watching out for the both of you and if you need me, just talk to me just like Mom and I talk to our Moms and Dads. They are always watching out for us."

Buddy asked "Do you promise meDad?" and I said "I promise Buddy and remember you will always be "My Best Friend"."

I also told him that we shouldn't worry about things that may or may not happen. We don't know how much time I will actually have left. I do know that when they do tell me it will be the saddest day of my life.

Then Buddy said, "Dad do you ever get scared?" and I replied "Yes I do, but that is normal and don't you ever tell Mom that I get scared." He looked at me and said "You don't have to worry about that Dad. I would never tell anyone any of our secrets."

So, I said to him. "Buddy, don't get upset about all of this, you just have to look at it like we do and that is one Cystoscopy at a time."

With tears in his eyes he just turned and looked at the trees and the sky without saying a word.

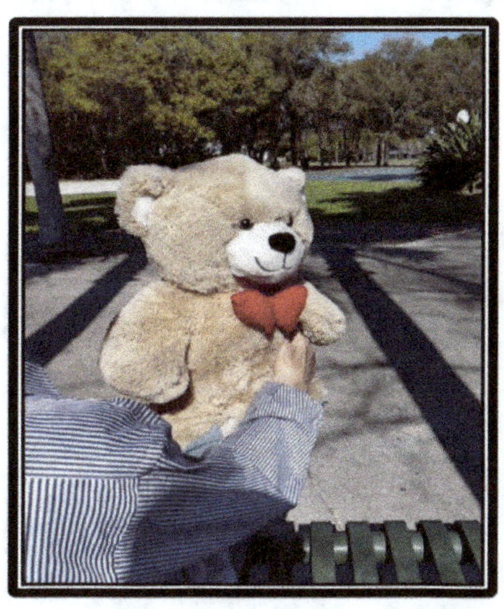

There was silence for a few moments. Then I said to Buddy "In my heart of hearts Buddy, I'm hoping to be around for several more years to come."

I also mentioned to him the choice is not ours to make, "it is the "luck of the draw" or the "higher powers" decision. It depends on how you believe and what you believe."

Buddy just kept staring at the
trees and the sky with tears in his eyes
and with his little gruff voice he said "I
love you Dad and I want to go home now."

So we did.

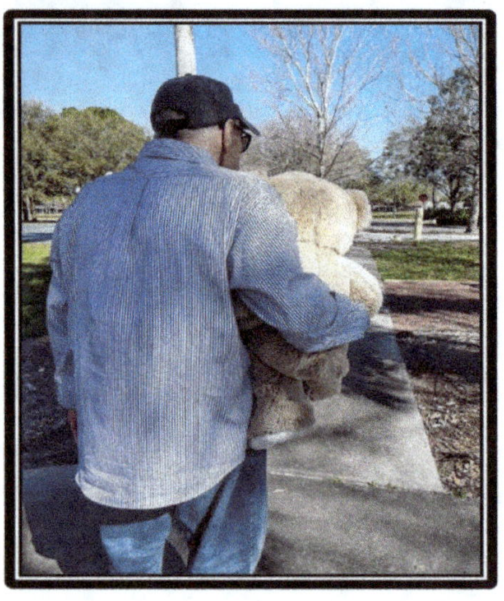

In closing, *I do have to tell you one extremely important factor that keeps this process in prospective for all that goes on whether it is Cancer, Dementia, Alzheimer's or any other life changing disease that is eventually going to kill you. ("Sorry for being so blunt")*

That important factor is your Caretaker. The mental and physical responsibility is so overwhelming and there will be many times it could be considered abusive.

Your Caretaker has to be determined, loving, caring, and patient beyond patience and let's not forget having to maintain a very large dose of understanding.

It would be a Mexican stand off to decide who has the better end of the deal and if your Caretaker is your spouse, you better love each other to the Moon and back.

Your spouse will be taking care of everything you ever did and would be doing now, as well as taking care of themselves.

Don't forget the entire household? "One person gets the job"!!!

There will be times that resentment will arise between the both of you and it won't be by choice. It is human nature regardless of how close the two of you are.

You will feel trapped and helpless at times and those feelings will probably be the most difficult of all to overcome.

It is a roller coaster ride of emotions for both of you. There will be a lot of laughter and twice as many tears that you will share together and alone.

As I had mentioned previously, Buddy was our "Distraction" and shortly thereafter became a part of our family. Everyone should experience the same joy as we have during a difficult time and it was all because of Buddy the Bear, "My Best Friend"

I would like for you to meet my Caretaker and my Wife. The moment I met her I knew I was going to marry her and I did.

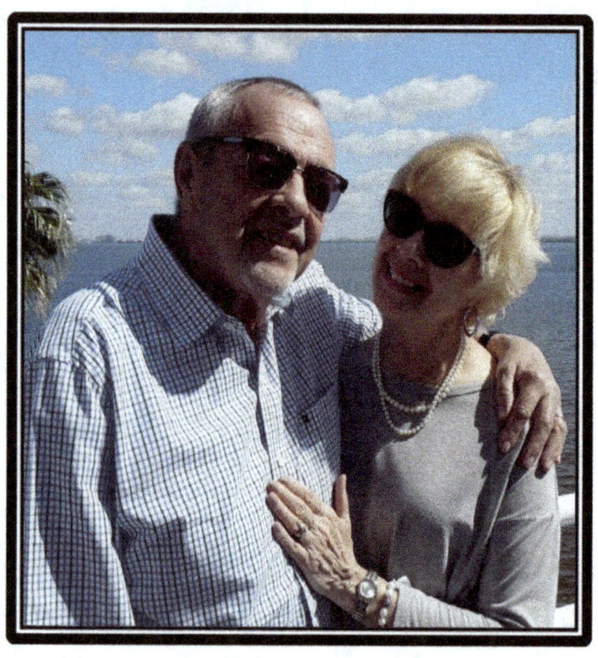

We renew our vows on our Anniversary every year to reaffirm our promise of respect, love, best friends forever and to always take care of each other. "I love her with all of my heart and my soul."